Hypothyroidism Diet

Natural Remedies And Foods To Boost Your Energy And Jump Start Your Weight Loss

By Susan T. Williams

This book is designed to provide information on the topic covered. The information herein is offered for informational purposes solely. It is sold with the understanding that neither the author nor the publisher is engaged in rendering legal, accounting or other professional services. If legal or other professional advice is warranted, the services of an appropriate professional should be sought.

While every effort has been made to make the information presented here as complete and accurate as possible, it may contain errors, omissions or information that was accurate as of its publication but subsequently has become outdated by marketplace or industry changes. Neither author nor publisher accepts any liability or responsibility to any person or entity with respect to any loss or damage alleged to have been caused, directly or indirectly, by the information, ideas, opinions or other content in this book.

In no way, is it legal to reproduce, duplicate, or transmit any part of this document in either electronic means or printed form. Recording of this publication is strictly prohibited and any storage of this document is not allowed unless with written permission from the publisher.

The use of any trademark within this book is for clarifying purposes only, and any trademarks referenced in this work are used are without consent, and remain the property of the respective trademark holders, who are not affiliated with the publisher or this book.

Table of Contents

Chapter 1: Hypothyroidism: The Basic Facts 1

Chapter 2: Causes and Symptoms of Hypothyroidism 3

Chapter 3: Risk factors and Complications 7

Chapter 4: Treatment and Management 9

Chapter 5: Thyroid Recipes and Meal Plans...15

  Breakfast Recipes 15

    Sweet Potato Waffles...15

    Fat-Burning Buttermilk Pancakes..16

    Simple Sandwich Bread Recipe 17

    Shredded Carrots and Beets with Scrambled Eggs...............................17

    Goji Grapefruit Parsley Smoothie 18

  Lunch Recipes 18

    Poached Salmon with Pumpkin Seed Parsley Sauce 18

    Turkey Pot Pie 20

    Arugula Salad with Salmon, Tomato and Avocado 21

    Sardine Salad Nicoise 21

    Roasted Sweet Potato Wedges...22

    Red Wine Chicken with Mushrooms 23

    Green Coconut Curry Mussels 24

    Fermented Fish Recipe...24

    Cucumber Avocado Summer Soup 25

    Chicken Liver 26

  Dinner Recipes..27

    Wild Rice Pilaf 27

    Brown Rice with Tomato and Avocado..27

    Lamb Burger with Kalamata Olives and Mint Gremolata 28

    German Rouladen 29

    Lima Bean Hummus 29

    Vegetable Soup...30

Instructions: 30

Slow Cooker Black Bean Soup 31

Thai Beef Salad..31

Herb Roasted Turkey Tenderloin...................................32

Lentil Stew 33

Conclusion...35

Introduction

Hypothyroidism is a condition that affects millions of people yet still goes under-diagnosed. This is because most of the symptoms associated with an under-active thyroid gland can also be attributed to other diseases, making correct diagnosis difficult.

Dealing with an underactive thyroid gland means that you have to deal with excessive weight gain and a lack of energy. Though there may be drugs and medicines out there for treating the condition, you can never go wrong with a hypothyroidism diet that provides natural remedies to boost your energy and help you shed those pounds.

If you open up any magazine, newspaper, or just switch on the TV, you will are sure to be bombarded by info about a new pill, supplement, or wonder cure on the market. Just as there are some medical experts who swear by these fads, there are others who oppose them. However, if there is one thing all experts agree on, it's that a natural and well balanced diet is one of the best ways to achieve optimal health.

What this means is that eating a variety of whole foods will provide your body with something that packaged and processed foods cannot. In fact, some of these natural nutrients are yet to be named by our so-called scientists – they know they are beneficial but haven't identified them yet! That is how powerful a natural balanced diet is to your overall health, especially when it comes to treating an underactive thyroid. But getting all the information you need about these natural diets and meal plans is not easy. That is where this book comes in.

This book is a treasure trove of proven strategies and recipes that are useful in the treatment and management of an under-active thyroid. In this book, you will get to understand the signs and symptoms of hypothyroidism, what causes the condition, and the myriad of natural foods that can help you fight the disease. If you have ever wondered how you are going to beat hypothyroidism and live a long and healthy life, then congratulations for picking up this book. You have taken the first step in the right direction.

I hope you enjoy the book!

CHAPTER 1

Hypothyroidism: The Basic Facts

In order to fully treat a disease, it is important that we fully understand what we are dealing with. So let us look at some basic facts that will help in understanding what hypothyroidism is.

So what exactly is hypothyroidism? This is a medical condition where a person's thyroid gland fails to produce enough thyroid hormones, specifically triodothyronine (T3) and thyroxine (T4). In other words, it is a flaw in the endocrine system, which is supposed to regulate the thyroid gland. The thyroid is a butterfly-shaped gland located right under the Adam's apple, and its main job is to produce hormones that regulate the metabolism.

Hypothyroidism can be attributed to one main cause – lack of iodine in the diet. This is a situation that is very common around the world, more so in developing countries. However, in countries where the diet contains sufficient quantities of iodine, the major cause of hypothyroidism is actually a condition referred to as 'chronic autoimmune thyroiditis' or Hashimoto's Thyroiditis. This is an auto-immune disease where your own immune cells attack and destroy your thyroid gland.

There are also other less-common causes of hypothyroidism that you should be aware of. These include pregnancies, problems with certain glands within the brain, thyroid removal surgeries, and trauma to the thyroid gland.

If you happen to be suffering from hypothyroidism, the first thing that you will notice is that your metabolism is really slow and you are constantly fatigued. When the disease strikes children, it typically leads to slow growth and poor intellectual development. The severity of the symptoms is usually an indication of just how advanced the hypothyroidism is.

It is also important to note that your body is dependent on the thyroid hormones for a number of other internal processes. What this means is that hypothyroidism does not just relate to your thyroid gland alone. There may be abnormalities in growth, cellular functions, and even mental development.

It is estimated that more than 27 million Americans are afflicted by thyroid diseases, and up to 13 million cases are undiagnosed. Almost three quarters of such thyroid disease cases are due to hypothyroidism. This is a stark and scary statistic. It means that there are millions of people out there who have no idea that they are suffering from this disease, and are probably taking pills for curing the symptoms instead of tackling the root cause.

The usual approach that most people take to beat this disease is medication. However, such medication is taken for your entire lifetime. Imagine spending your whole life popping L-thyroxine pills every day, just so that your Thyroid Stimulating Hormones (TSH) can be maintained at a normal level.

However, you need to know that there are natural ways of controlling hypothyroidism, and this book is dedicated to showing you just how to do that.

CHAPTER 2

Causes and Symptoms of Hypothyroidism

Now that we have looked at the general facts about hypothyroidism, let's move on to the causes of the disease and the signs and symptoms to keep an eye out for.

The causes of hypothyroidism are usually grouped into two categories — primary and secondary causes.

Primary Causes

Primary causes are those that occur inside the thyroid gland itself. A good example is thyroid autoimmunity, which is a situation where the immune system produces antibodies that attack the thyroid gland. This is the major cause of hypothyroidism in the western world.

Thyroid autoimmunity causes severe damage to the thyroid tissue as time goes by, ultimately resulting in an underactive thyroid. However, it doesn't stop there. Whatever normal thyroid tissue you have left is soon replaced by abnormal tissue. So what difference does that make to your thyroid function?

Well, the iodine that is contained in all the food you eat cannot be absorbed by the abnormal tissue. Only the normal healthy tissue can do this. This practically starves your thyroid gland of iodine that is vital for producing the thyroid hormone. Apart from that, the abnormal tissue forms tiny tumors which occupy a lot of space inside the gland, virtually preventing the remaining normal tissue from functioning properly.

There are also other primary causes of hypothyroidism. These include physical trauma to the thyroid gland (for example during a car crash) and immature development of the thyroid gland at birth.

Secondary Causes

Secondary causes can be described as those that occur elsewhere inside the body but still indirectly affect the level of thyroid hormones. For example, there could be a chemical ingredient that the thyroid requires for proper functioning but the body cannot provide it. This is what happens in cases where there is not enough iodine in the diet. The hypothyroidism develops because the thyroid cannot produce hormones for regulating metabolism without the all-important iodine.

There are also cases where the thyroid gland is damaged by toxic chemicals, say in areas where the source of drinking water has been polluted by radioactive material.

In female patients, an underactive thyroid could be the result of what is known as 'postpartum hypothyroidism', which is a condition where the thyroid fails to function properly after pregnancy.

So why is it important for you to understand the cause of your hypothyroidism? It is crucial that every hypothyroidism patient understands the cause of their condition because different individuals will have different triggers for the condition. You may find yourself comparing your treatment with another person who also suffers from an underactive thyroid, yet the underlying causes of your condition may be different.

In order to better manage your treatment as an individual, you should ask your doctor to diagnose the specific cause(s) of your hypothyroidism. Though it may require some extra diagnostic tests, it will eventually help you become more knowledgeable about the condition affecting you.

Signs and Symptoms

When it comes to hypothyroidism, the symptoms that result from the disease tend to manifest themselves in different ways. Here are some of the most common symptoms to look out for, in case you are not sure whether you have the disease or not.
Aching muscles and joints
Dry skin
Depression
Edema, or swelling in the body
Weight gain
Loss of hair
Fatigue and lack of energy
Water retention
Constipation
An increase in cholesterol levels
Slow breathing and reduced pulse rate
Goiter
Menstrual cycles that are heavier than normal
Change in appetite
If you look at some of these symptoms closely, you will see that they mimic those of senility and even Alzheimer's disease. The moment the disease is treated, however, most of the symptoms that were assumed to be due to old age are reversed.

Diagnosis

Diagnosing a disease such as hypothyroidism requires you to visit a medical specialist. It is important that you get the opinion of a trained medical professional whenever you are suffering from any of the symptoms that we talked about previously. This way, you can receive a proper diagnosis as to the cause of your condition.

When you walk into the doctor's office for a checkup, they will initially ask about the symptoms you are exhibiting as well as your family's medical history. This information is crucial because it helps the doctor to assess your condition and whether you have any risk factors for hypothyroidism.

You will also undergo some kind of physical assessment that may reveal the presence of an enlarged thyroid, dry skin, large tongue or slow reflexes. These are used as indicators of the development of hypothyroidism.

These are just the preliminary tests that you will likely have to undergo. However, the majority of hypothyroidism cases are diagnosed via laboratory blood tests. What the doctor does is to order what is known as a thyroid panel (multiple tests) or simply a single test. The tests are meant to measure the levels of T3 and T4 hormones you have in your thyroid, and also the levels of TSH (thyroid stimulating hormone) in your blood.

A positive determination of hypothyroidism is made if your levels of TSH are elevated and your levels of T3 and/or T4 are low. An elevated level of TSH is regarded as a sign that your thyroid gland is unable to produce this hormone in sufficient quantities, thus forcing your pituitary gland to step in and give it an abnormally high boost.

At the end of the day, a proper diagnosis is what will make the difference between treating the actual root cause of hypothyroidism and simply managing the individual symptoms.

CHAPTER 3

Risk factors and Complications

There are some factors that put you more at risk of developing hypothyroidism. These factors have been proven to contribute to an underactive thyroid gland, and in this chapter we try to understand what they are and how they affect you. Diseases that affect the balance of thyroid hormones can affect anybody and at any point in life. However, there are specific genetic factors and other natural situations that place some individuals at higher risk of developing hypothyroidism. Check out the factors listed below and how they affect you.

Being Female

If you are a woman, then your risk of developing an underactive thyroid goes up five times. In other words, hypothyroidism is five times more common in females than in males. But why is this so?

The simple answer is that women have more complex endocrine systems than men. The endocrine system is what is responsible for producing hormones, and we all know that the female body tends to produce a diverse range of hormones. The work of these hormones is to regulate everything from the menstrual cycle to the process of giving birth.

Such fertility and reproductive cycles result in wide variations in the levels of thyroid, adrenal, and sex hormones, which is probably why females are more likely to suffer from hormonal imbalances of the endocrine system.

In order to understand this better, try to visualize the endocrine system as a loop. Since the system works in unison, variations in the levels of a particular hormone will ultimately affect the levels of the rest of the other hormones.

There is also a possibility that such hormonal changes trigger the immune system of some women to produce antibodies which then attack the glands causing wide variations in hormone levels. In cases where the thyroid gland is affected, 'thyroid autoimmunity' develops. When women approach menopause, their reproductive response becomes slow, also contributing to an imbalance in the thyroid hormone.

Having an autoimmune disease

In the event that you are already suffering from another autoimmune disease, then your chances of developing hypothyroidism go up. Diseases such as pernicious anemia, rheumatoid arthritis, Sjogrens syndrome, type 1 diabetes, and lupus are all risk factors of thyroid gland diseases.

Genetic Factors

Did any of your parents or grandparents suffer from hypothyroidism? If you answered yes to this question, then you are at greater risk of developing the disease too.

Being pregnant

If you are pregnant or have given birth within the last six months, then your risk of developing hypothyroidism goes up. However, I must state that fewer than ten percent of women actually end up developing postpartum thyroiditis. For those women that do become affected, the condition usually resolves itself without any treatment, so there is no need to fear. Treatment only becomes necessary in cases where the hypothyroidism recurs.

Ethnicity

Research has shown that Caucasians tend to suffer from more cases of hypothyroidism than African-Americans.

I want you to keep in mind that you may develop hypothyroidism with or without the risk factors highlighted above. Just because you satisfy the conditions doesn't mean you will automatically get the disease. On the other hand, the likelihood of developing an underactive thyroid gland goes up depending on the number of risk factors you have.

CHAPTER 4

Treatment and Management

Treating and managing hypothyroidism in an effective manner requires you to change your lifestyle. You will have to carefully consider what you eat and how you exercise.

As we have seen in the previous chapters, one of the many symptoms of an under-active thyroid is an increase in weight due to the slowing down of your metabolism. When your metabolism becomes sluggish, you naturally stop burning calories as fast as you used to. This means that you may be eating the same amount of food as before, or maybe even less, but your weight just keeps going up. This can be exacerbated further by other hypothyroid effects such as water retention, increased cholesterol and fatigue, which make it even more difficult for you to shed those pounds.

If your thyroid problem is the result of autoimmune thyroiditis, then it will probably be harder for you to lose the weight, even after your hormone levels have gone back to normal. Medical specialists still don't know why this is the case, but the common assumption is that it is due to resistance to insulin or variations in brain chemistry.

Since hypothyroidism is something that you have to contend with for the rest of your life, it goes without saying that you have to manage the symptoms if you truly want to feel better. This can only be done when you embrace a healthy all-natural diet and get plenty of exercise.

From my experience with hypothyroidism, there are certain realities that you will have to face up to sooner or later. Though you may drop a few pounds, it is highly unlikely that you will go back to the size you once were. Another thing is that you may not be able to lose weight as fast as you did before, or as fast as other people do. These are things you have to bear in mind, and though it may be tough to accept at first, it will ultimately help you to be realistic about your weight loss goals and objectives.

Living with hypothyroidism is not easy, but you can live a normal and happy life if you focus on other important stuff. Instead of trying to attain a specific weight or size, my advice would be to focus on boosting your energy levels and reducing those feelings of depression and fatigue that you will constantly be battling. This will ultimately improve your quality of life.

With that said, let us take a look at what your average hypothyroid diet looks like.

The Hypothyroid Diet

To follow a hypothyroidism diet, the first thing to do is to consume foods that are a good source of tyrosine. Tyrosine is an amino acid that combines well with iodine to aid the production of thyroid hormones. So go for foods like fish, bananas, dairy, almonds, oats, avocados, and sesame seeds.

Another thing you must do is reduce your carbohydrate intake. Studies have shown that people with hypothyroidism should have only 45 - 50% of their total calorie intake from carbohydrates. The rest of your diet should be made up of about 30% protein and 20% fat. On the other hand, a large part of your carb intake should be from complex carbohydrates such as fresh veggies, fruits, and whole grains (whole wheat pasta and bread, wheat germ and brown rice). Complex carbs are more nutritious for you than the refined kind, and are full of zinc and B vitamins.

We all know that too much sugar is bad for you, but for a person living with hypothyroidism, sugar can be terrible for your condition. Avoid sugar laden foods such as chips, cookies, candy, pies, cake, ice cream and the like. Do not forget that if you are going to cook using salt, make sure it is the iodized kind.

Most of the stuff we eat nowadays is packed with carbohydrates, so it's normal to find yourself sitting down to a meal or snack that is composed of pure carbs. However, this is not something that is recommended for hypothyroid patients. You have to add some protein into the meal, the reason being that protein is digested slowly by the body, thus slowing down the production of insulin. Sea food, eggs, shellfish, meat and dairy are great sources of protein and are recommended for hypothyroid sufferers who need to maintain their weight. In fact, these are also great sources of vitamin B12 and zinc.

Hypothyroidism comes with a lethargic digestion process. Unfortunately, this is also followed by constipation. However, if you increase your intake of fiber to about 30 to 40 grams daily, you can help your system speed things up a bit. Another benefit of fiber, as you well know, is that it keeps you full for longer. You can therefore kill two birds with one stone.

There are a variety of minerals and vitamins that can provide your thyroid with the nourishment it needs to maintain healthy function. These include the anti-oxidizing vitamins E, C and A; vitamins B12, B6, B3 and B2; and zinc. You should stock up on things like olive oil, nuts, whole grains, and whole wheat bread so that you can get your healthy dose of B vitamins. Raw herbs like parsley should also be incorporated into meals as a garnish due to their high vitamin C content.

If there is one piece of advice that you should never ever ignore, it's this — drink enough water every day. There is no substitute for a glass of water. Some people may rather drink fresh juice, but that's not good enough. You need 8 to 12 cups of H2O daily if you want to keep your already sluggish metabolism working at optimal level. You should switch to using purified water for both drinking and cooking because regular water contains fluoride — which has been discovered to interfere with thyroid function.

Remember, part of your treatment requires you to exercise, so you need to replace the water you have lost via sweating. And now that you are consuming more fiber, water becomes even more essential.

What Foods to Avoid

So far we have talked about what to do and eat in terms of a healthy diet, but there are also certain foods that can do more harm than good.

There is a class of naturally occurring substances, known as goitrogens, which tend to interfere with thyroid hormone production. These are the same hormones that hypothyroid sufferers already lack, so you can see how goitrogens can be a problem. Goitrogens can be found in specific foods which, unfortunately, are quite popular within the health-food community. Think of broccoli, cabbage, kale, peanuts, millet, spinach, cauliflower, peaches, and soybeans - all these foods are great sources of tyrosine, but they also contain goitrogens.

Some health specialists are of the opinion that these goitrogens can be inactivated when food is cooked, so make sure that you cook these foods well before you eat them. Another thing you need to know about foods containing goitrogens is that they may be healthy for you, but you have to consider their goitrogenic potential. This should especially concern people who are regarded as at-risk: women close to menopause, people already exhibiting hypothyroid symptoms and people with a hereditary predisposition to the condition.

You should also try to avoid drinking stimulants. Yes, I realize how difficult this one might be, but you'll be better off for it. When you feel like your energy levels are starting to dip, its normal for most people to reach for that cup of tea, coffee or soda, but these foods will only weaken your adrenal system further. An under-active thyroid overworks the adrenal glands, and downing cup after cup of stimulants will result in burnout of the adrenal system. The bottom line is – heal your adrenal system by weaning yourself off of stimulants.

Hypothyroidism and Exercise

One of the biggest problems that a hypothyroidism sufferer will face is uncontrollable weight gain. You can easily find yourself 20 pounds over your normal weight, but this is not due to the condition itself. The cause is actually the feeling of fatigue that takes over your life. You feel tired all the time and as a result, working out becomes the last thing on your mind. The lack of exercise then causes your body to feel even more fatigued, thus turning the situation into a vicious cycle. The fact of the matter is, if you want to truly lose weight and eliminate fatigue, then exercise is key to achieving your goals.

So what are some of the best forms of exercise that you can perform for hypothyroidism? Well, you can start with some low-impact aerobic workouts and some strength training. Aerobic exercises get your heart pumping and your lungs going without running the risk of stressing out your joints, because we know that joint pain is one symptom of hypothyroidism. You can take up yoga or Pilates to boost your core muscles or you may even get yourself an elliptical machine or stationary bike to enhance your cardio health.

When it comes to strength training, there are many options available to you. If pumping iron is your thing, then you will benefit from lifting weights. If you prefer something less strenuous, then you can perform leg raises, lunges or pushups. The crucial thing to remember is that strength training leads to an increase in muscle mass, and muscle burns more calories than fat. What this means is that having more muscle can help prevent the weight gain that is associated with hypothyroidism.

Having said that, it's time we examined in detail some of the recommended exercises for people with an underactive thyroid:

Pushups – Place both palms on the ground, shoulder width apart. Stretch your feet out behind you and keep them together. Then bend your elbows and lower yourself as close to the floor as possible, before coming back up. If you feel this is too hard, then perform the pushup with your hands on a table or wall and your feet on the floor.
Squats – Stand upright and then slowly bend at the knees until you find yourself in a sitting position. Return to the starting position and repeat.

One-legged dead lift – Balance yourself on one leg as you support yourself by holding onto something. Place one hand gently in front of your thigh. Keep your back straight. Then push your hips backwards as far as possible, until your hand reaches the floor. Return to your original position. This move works the glutes as well.

Lap pull-down – Using an overhand grip, get hold of a pull-down bar. Raise yourself up until the bar reaches your collar bone. Ensure that your spine remains straight as you do this.

Overhead press – Grab a pair of dumbbells and bring them to shoulder height. Rotate your arms so that the palms face forward. Raise the dumbbells up, keeping your elbows straight. Lower the weights back down to shoulder height.

For aerobic exercises, the general recommendation is 3 to 4 times every week. For strength training, you should go for 2 to 3 days every week. Please remember that you have to consult your doctor before you start any exercise routine. Also keep in mind that working out can never be a replacement for thyroid medication.

Benefits of Exercise

For a person with an underactive thyroid, exercise can have immense benefits. Outlined below are some of the advantages you get from sticking with an exercise regimen:

People with hypothyroidism tend to have low serotonin levels, which leads to depression, poor sleep patterns and lack of appetite control. Half an hour of aerobic exercise performed 5 times every week can boost your serotonin levels and help avoid such symptoms.

Exercise helps to minimize stress, which is one of the major causes of overeating. The adrenal glands are responsible for stress reactions, and since theses glands are malfunctioning in hypothyroid patients, they are unable to regulate stress.

Exercise helps to boost your metabolism, which is something every hypothyroid patient needs. So get moving, and you will begin to feel more energetic.

The deep breathing that comes with exercise and yoga helps in taking in more oxygen, which is great for reducing stress, losing weight, and general relaxation.

As we end this chapter, I would like you to keep the following things in mind whenever you are setting your dietary and exercise goals:

Hypothyroidism is a lifelong condition, so your lifestyle will have to change. There can be no substitute for a healthy natural diet, exercising and loving yourself. Reading this book means that you are starting off in the right direction, but you have to stay committed to changing your lifestyle.

Always stay optimistic, and don't forget to recognize the positives in your new lifestyle, be they large or small. You should take up journaling as a way to note the high and low points of your journey, as this is what will keep you going during those low and frustrating periods.

Keep your eyes focused on the goal. It may seem like change is not happening quickly enough for your liking, but those small baby steps will eventually get you where you want to go. Just do your best everyday and if you ever stumble, pick yourself up, dust yourself off, and keep moving forward.

Nothing good ever comes easy, so do not be swayed by new health or weigh loss fads when it comes to managing hypothyroidism. Remember the saying, 'if it's too good to be true'.

CHAPTER 5

Thyroid Recipes and Meal Plans

If you consider yourself a foodie, then you're going to love this chapter. There are many different recipes and meal plans provided here, and they are all natural and healthy remedies for an underactive thyroid. The recipes have been categorized into breakfast, lunch and dinner recipes. Enjoy!

Breakfast Recipes

Sweet Potato Waffles

This is a simple and healthy choice for breakfast that does not take long to whip up. You can make it over the weekend and store it in the refrigerator; just toast it and you're ready to go.

Ingredients:

1 cup egg whites
½ tsp Celtic sea salt
1 tsp baking soda
1 roasted organic sweet potato, medium sized
8 tbsp organic coconut flour

5 tbsp organic coconut milk
4 pastured eggs
20 drops SweetLeaf Stevia Clear Liquid Stevia
½ tsp organic cinnamon
4 pastured eggs

Instructions:

1. Take a medium-sized bowl, and place the coconut milk, Stevia, egg whites, sweet potato and eggs into it. Blend the mixture into a smooth mix using an immersion blender. Alternatively, you can use a blender.

2. Place the dry ingredients (cinnamon, salt, baking soda, and coconut flour) in a bowl and whisk them.
3. Add the dry ingredients to the smooth mix in the first bowl, and blend together at high speed.
4. Take your cast iron waffle pan (PFTE/PFOA free iron), and spray it with coconut oil. Then preheat the waffle pan.
5. Use a ladle to scoop ¼ to ½ a cup of the mixture onto the iron waffle pan, cover the pan, and cook for about one minute. The cooking time may vary depending on the temperature settings.
6. Serve the dish with butter and some sugar-free maple syrup.

Serves: 6

Fat-Burning Buttermilk Pancakes

Pancakes may seem like an indulgent and unhealthy way to start off your day, but this dish is quite different. They are not like your conventional buttermilk pancakes that come in a box or the "organic" ones you buy from the store. These are dairy free, grain free and gluten free pancakes packed with protein, fiber, selenium and vitamin B12; ingredients that are naturally suited for treating thyroid problems. Go ahead and enjoy this nutrient –rich breakfast!

Ingredients:

1 tsp baking soda
½ cup coconut buttermilk
½ cup coconut flour
2 tsp cinnamon

6 pastured eggs
8-10 drops Clear Liquid Stevia
1 tbsp coconut nectar

Instructions:

1. Place the coconut buttermilk, coconut nectar, and eggs in a blender. Blend the mixture well.
2. Add the cinnamon, baking soda, and coconut flour into the blender and mix until smooth.
3. Allow the blended mixture to rest for 5 minutes.
4. Take an enameled cast-iron griddle (non-stick) and heat it to medium heat. Pour the batter into the pan in silver dollar-size amounts. Cook the pancakes for one minute before flipping. You can continue making more batches of batter.
5. Serve with organic frozen blueberry sauce and Kerrygold butter.

Serves: 4(yields 16-20 small pancakes).

Simple Sandwich Bread Recipe

This breakfast recipe is easy to make and is perfect for busy people who don't have time to sit down and have a large breakfast in the morning. You can prepare it the night before and store it for the next day. The meal contains no gluten, dairy, or grains. On top of that, it is low in carbs, which is great if you want to lose weight.

Ingredients:

4 large pastured eggs   ½ tsp Celtic sea salt
12 tbsp organic coconut flour   ½ cup melted organic butter

Instructions:

1. Preheat the oven to 350° F.
2. Take a 9 inch by 5 inch loaf pan and grease the surface.
3. Combine all the ingredients in a medium-sized bowl and mix thoroughly.
4. Pour the mixture into the loaf pan.
5. Bake for about 40 minutes.
6. Place the loaf on a cooling rack to let it cool before serving.

Serves: 12

Shredded Carrots and Beets with Scrambled Eggs

If you are the kind of person who loves raw vegetables but is tired of eating the same old lettuce over and over, then this recipe is just for you. It's healthy, easy to make, and can be served with a range of other foods. You can decide to substitute the eggs with something like ground beef and convert it to a light lunch dish.

Ingredients:

3 golden beets   3 tbsp white or apple cider vinegar
5 carrots   Pepper
4 organic eggs   Real sea salt
6 fresh or dried thyme sprigs

Instructions:

1. Firstly, peel the carrots and beets.
2. Shred the carrots and beets using either a Cuisinart or by hand.
3. Mix the carrots and beets in a bowl and toss with the thyme and vinegar. You can add the salt and pepper to taste.

4. Set aside and refrigerate.
5. Prepare the scrambled eggs and serve with the carrot/beet salad.

Serves: 2

Goji Grapefruit Parsley Smoothie

This is a breakfast meal that gives your body and thyroid energy as well as blood-balance. Goji berries (also known as wolf berries) contain iron, selenium, vitamin C, zinc and riboflavin (B2). These are some of the key elements that are used in treating thyroid patients. The parsley and grapes are thrown in to help in liver detoxification, which is vital for good thyroid nutrition.

Ingredients:

1 grapefruit
1 handful of hemp seeds
1 handful of dry goji berries
1 handful of fresh parsley

1 cup filtered water
1 tbsp milk thistle
1 ½ ground flax seeds
1 handful of walnuts, pecans or almonds

Instructions:

1. Soak the goji berries in water overnight or at least two hours before using them. You can re-use this water to later make your smoothie.
2. Put all the ingredients above in a blender.
3. Blend to a smooth consistency, depending on how smooth or chunky you like your smoothie.
4. Enjoy your smoothie!

Serves: 1

Lunch Recipes

Poached Salmon with Pumpkin Seed Parsley Sauce

Poached salmon is an excellent source of vitamin B12, which provides the body with additional energy while keeping the nervous system healthy. The parsley offers a healthy dose of vitamin C and beta-carotene, while the pumpkin seeds are full of tyrosine.

Pumpkin seed parsley sauce ingredients:

1 clove garlic, peeled

1 cup fresh parsley, coarsely chopped

1 cup raw pumpkin seeds

1 ½ Parmesan cheese, freshly grated

2 tbsp cold-pressed olive oil

4 tsp lemon juice, freshly squeezed

1 tsp iodized salt

Poached salmon ingredients:

1 ½ pounds salmon fillet

2 tbsp white wine vinegar

1 bay leaf

1 tsp iodized salt

4 fresh thyme sprigs

Instructions:

1. The sauce should be prepared first. Drop the garlic into a running food processor. Stop the processor, scrape down the sides, and then pour the cheese, seeds, and parsley into the processor. Re-start the processor and steadily pour the olive oil through the feed tube. Switch off the processor once more, and scrape the sides. Stir the mixture and process again. Once this is done, scoop the sauce into a bowl and add lemon juice and salt. Stir the mixture well.

2. Pour fresh water in a deep pan, enough to immerse the salmon. Add the thyme, bay leaf, salt, and vinegar to the pan, and boil the water. Keep the heat medium-low and the pan uncovered, and make sure to watch the water.

3. Once the water begins quivering, measure the thickest section of the fish before placing it into the pan. The fish is to be cooked 7 - 8 minutes for every inch of thickness. When the salmon is half-done, pour some of the fish water into the sauce mixture and stir.

4. Pour ¾ of the pumpkin seed parsley sauce into a warm serving platter. Confirm whether the thickest section of the fish is well cooked; if the fillet is opaque and springs back when pressed with a fork, then it's ready. Put the fish on top of the sauce, and pour the left over sauce over the fish in a decorative manner.

Serves: 4

Turkey Pot Pie

Ingredients:

1 thinly sliced organic carrot, medium-sized

1 ½ cups chicken broth

½ tsp freshly ground black pepper

1 organic onion, chopped

3 tbsp organic shortening

3 eight oz. pasture-bred chicken breasts, diced into one-inch chunks

2 oz. sliced organic white button mushrooms

1 large pasture-raised egg

2 tbsp freshly chopped parsley

1 cup organic coconut milk

¾ teaspoon Celtic sea salt

2 organic celery stalks, thinly sliced

½ tbsp organic arrowroot

1 tsp baking soda

½ tsp dried savory

1 ½ cups ground organic almond flour

1 tsp dried thyme

Instructions:

1. Start by making the dough. Mix the baking soda, salt and almond flour in a medium-sized bowl. Add the shortening and rub it into the flour using your fingers; continue until the mixture looks like coarse sand. Beat the egg in a bowl and add it into the mix, kneading the dough with your hands until it's all moist. Cool the dough in a refrigerator for a quarter of an hour.

2. Take the chicken pieces, mushrooms, broth, carrot, onions, and celery and place them in a medium sauce pot. Bring the mixture to a boil, and then put in the herbs. Lower the heat and simmer for fifteen minutes, until the veggies are tender and the chicken is well done.

3. Preheat the oven to 350° F.

4. Sieve the stock into a saucepan, add the coconut milk, and bring to a boil. Pour two tablespoons of cold water into a small cup and add in the arrowroot. Stir the mixture well before pouring it into the saucepan with the stock. Whisk the mixture and cook for two minutes until it thickens.

5. Pour the thick sauce over the veggies and chicken pieces, making sure to coat everything. Add the parsley and season with pepper and salt.

6. Take the dough out of the refrigerator. Place one sheet of unbleached parchment paper underneath and another over the dough. Roll it a quarter to half an inch thick. You can make single pot pies using eight-ounce ramekins or a nine-inch pot pie.

7. Use a spoon to scoop the chicken and veggie fillings into a pie pan. Cut the dough into suitable sizes and lay over the fillings. Use the tines of a fork to press down the edges of the dough to stick to the pie pan rim.

8. Bake for 25 to 30 minutes until the dough turns golden brown and is a bit puffy. If the edges of the dough brown too fast, cover them with aluminum foil.
9. Serve.

Serves: 6

Arugula Salad with Salmon, Tomato and Avocado

Ingredients:

1 organic tomato, medium size, diced into chunks

2 tbsp organic extra virgin olive oil

2 cans Alaskan sockeye salmon

1 tsp honey

2 tbsp organic balsamic vinegar

1 sliced organic avocado

6 cups arugula

4 organic radishes, thinly sliced

1 organic red onion, thinly sliced

½ tsp Celtic sea salt

¼ tsp freshly ground black pepper

Instructions:

1. Drain the fish and separate it into chunks.
2. Pour the oil, honey, salt, balsamic vinegar, and pepper into a small bowl and whisk them together.
3. Divide the arugula into separate bowls and add a topping of onion, tomato, radishes, avocado and the chunks of salmon.
4. Apply the dressing.
5. Serve.

Serves: 4

Sardine Salad Nicoise

This salad is a deliciously nutritious dish that serves up all the natural ingredients for treating an underactive thyroid, including iodine. With a total preparation time of 35 minutes, the sardine salad nicoise is a dish you can make in no time at all.

Ingredients:

2 cups organic mixed greens

2 cans sardines

16 organic black olives

6 tbsp extra virgin olive oil

½ tsp Celtic sea salt

16 organic grape tomatoes

2 organic eggs

½ organic small red onion

½ tsp freshly ground black pepper

4 tbsp organic red wine vinegar

2 cups organic green beans

2 tsp organic Dijon mustard

Instructions:

1. Put the eggs in a saucepan, cover them in one inch of cold water, and boil over medium heat. Do not forget to cover the pan with a lid.
2. Once the water boils fully, remove the pan from the heat and let the eggs stay in the water for about 15 minutes.
3. Drain the hot water from the pan, and then add cold water and ice cubes into the pan with the eggs.
4. Meanwhile, place the green bean in a non-stick skillet and sauté them for about 3 minutes. Sauté just enough to turn the beans crispy and tender, and then set aside.
5. Take the eggs, remove the shells and slice them. Then put them aside.
6. Using a whisk, mix the mustard and vinegar together in a large bowl.
7. Gently drizzle the olive oil into the mixture and whisk until it thickens slightly.
8. Add salt and pepper to season.
9. Place the mixed greens in serving plates.
10. Top off with the egg slices, onion, green beans, sardines, and tomatoes.
11. Drizzle the dressing and then add the olives.

Serves: 4

Roasted Sweet Potato Wedges

This is a truly mouth-watering addition to your thyroid diet. In fact, once you start cooking your own chips and wedges, you'll never go back to another fast food restaurant for fries again. This is one dish your kids will love, so get them to help out with lunch on weekends. Enjoy!

Ingredients:

4 sweet potatoes, medium sized

2 tbsp coconut oil

Sea salt and pepper to taste

Ras El Hanout, a Moroccan spice
(optional)

Thyme, cumin or oregano

Instructions:

1. Preheat oven to 425° F.
2. Cut the sweet potatoes into wedges.
3. Mix the coconut oil, herbs, sea salt, and pepper in a bowl.

4. Toss the sweet potatoes with the mixture.
5. Spread the potato wedges out on parchment paper, making sure that they are not in contact with each other.
6. Bake for 45 minutes. Don't forget to turn them 2 to 3 times.
7. If you want the wedges to turn out crispy, you can leave the oven door slightly open.

Serves: 4

Red Wine Chicken with Mushrooms

Ingredients:

½ tsp Celtic sea salt
2 tbsp organic butter
1 tbsp organic avocado oil
½ tsp freshly ground black pepper
1 cup dry red wine
4 pasture-raised chicken legs

4 organic shallots
1 tbsp organic marjoram
1 tbsp organic tomato paste
8 ounces organic button mushrooms
2 cups organic chicken broth

Instructions:

1. Separate the chicken legs into drumsticks and thighs, then pat them dry.
2. Use the salt and pepper to season the chicken pieces.
3. Put the butter in a large stock pot and place over medium heat.
4. Place the chicken in the pot and remove when it begins to brown. Set them aside on a plate.
5. Finely chop the shallots and sauté them in the pot for five minutes over medium heat.
6. Add tomato paste into the pot and cook for one more minute.
7. Pour the wine in and raise the heat to high. Let the wine boil for about five minutes, until its level reduces by half.
8. Quarter the mushrooms, and toss them into the pot together with the chicken pieces and chicken broth.
9. Decrease the heat to low, partially cover the pot and let it simmer for 45 minutes. Wait until the chicken is well cooked and the sauce becomes thick.
10. Chop up the marjoram and stir into the pot.
11. Serve.

Serves: 4

Green Coconut Curry Mussels

Ingredients:

1 tbsp virgin coconut oil

1 ½ tbsp organic curry powder

3 tsp organic ginger

1 organic yellow onion

1 organic lime

½ cup chicken broth

Sea salt to taste

2 tbsp chopped cilantro

2 cups organic coconut milk

1 stalk lemongrass, cut and smashed

1/3 tsp red chili pepper

2 pounds New Zealand green-lipped mussels

Instructions:

1. Heat the coconut oil in a large pan. Then chop and sauté the onions until they turn soft and a bit translucent. Throw in the curry powder, minced ginger and chili. Stir the mixture for 1 minute.
2. Add the chicken broth. Let it simmer until it reduces to half.
3. Pour in the coconut milk, lemongrass and salt, and then increase the heat.
4. Place the mussels into the pan and lower the heat to medium. Cook for 6 to 7 minutes with the pan covered tight. Please note that frozen green-lipped mussels are bought already open, so if you are using fresh mussels, cook them until they open. Any mussels that refuse to open should be discarded.
5. Scoop the mussels into bowls, and garnish with juice from the lime wedges and chopped cilantro.
6. Serve.

Serves: 4

Fermented Fish Recipe

Eating fermented foods has a lot of benefits for overall health. Fermented foods are rich in beneficial bacteria, so this dish provides a great supply of nutrients for those with hypothyroidism.

Ingredients:

2 large and fresh mackerel or herring

1 cup Kefir whey

1 onion

1 tsp coriander seeds

2 tbsp sea salt per liter of brine

Fresh dill seeds

1 tbsp peppercorns

6 bay leaves

1 glass jar

Instructions:

1. Remove the skin and large bones from the fish, and chop into bite-size chunks.
2. Peel and cut the onion.
3. Put the coriander seeds, dill seeds, onion slices, peppercorns and bay leaves into the glass jar. Then toss the fish pieces into the jar and mix.
4. Take another jug, pour in some water and dissolve one tablespoon of sea salt. Pour in ½ cup of kefir whey into the jug.
5. Pour the brine from the jug into the glass jar, making sure that the fish pieces are fully covered. Make more brine if the fish is still uncovered.
6. Seal the jar tightly and let it ferment at room temperature for three to five days. After that, you can store it in the refrigerator.
7. You can serve the fish with fresh dill, mayonnaise, veggies, and spring onions.
8. Make sure you consume within one to three weeks.

Serves: 4

Cucumber Avocado Summer Soup

If there is one vegetable that makes the perfect meal on a hot summer day, then the cucumber would have to be it. Cucumbers are light, refreshing, and can be bulked up with avocados to create a sumptuous meal. With many veggies being off the table for most thyroid patients, it's great to find a vegetable that provides you with the antioxidants and anti-inflammatory properties necessary for a healthy thyroid. Let's take a look at how you can prepare this cool dish for a hot summer lunch.

Ingredients:

1 ripe avocado	1 lemon (use the skin zest and juice)
1 ½ pounds Persian cucumber	Chopped almonds
½ bunch freshly chopped mint	Fruity green olive oil
2 cloves garlic, chopped	1 tbsp freshly ground cumin
½ bunch chopped coriander	1 tsp sea salt

Instructions:

1. You don't have to peel the cucumbers, unless the skin is very tough
2. Put all the ingredients (except the avocado, olive oil and almonds) into a food processor and blend everything together until you get a smooth mixture.
3. Chop the avocado into chunks and throw them into the food processor. Continue blending until very smooth.

4. Place the blended mix into a bowl and chill it for a few hours. This allows the flavors to merge.
5. Serve the meal into plates and drizzle each serving with the olive oil. Then top it off with almonds.
6. Bon appétit!

Serves: 4

Chicken Liver

Chicken liver is one awesome source of vitamin A, vitamin B, RDA, iron and selenium. These are essential elements in every healthy thyroid diet. So instead of reaching for the vitamin and iron pills, just settle for a delicious meal of chicken liver. Please remember to avoid eating this meal with foods rich in calcium (e.g. cheese, yogurt or milk) as they tend to inhibit absorption of iron. You'd be better off eating it with foods laden with vitamin C (e.g. broccoli).

Ingredients:

½ pound chicken livers
2 bay leaves
1 tsp ground coriander
½ pound mushrooms
2 tbsp balsamic vinegar
3 tbsp olive or coconut oil
½ inch ginger root, grated
2 tsp ground cumin

½ tbsp lemon juice
2 garlic cloves, crushed
½ tsp red pepper, crushed
Pinch of salt
1 tbsp grass-fed butter
1 tbsp Sherry
1 tbsp Worcestershire sauce
1 onion

Instructions:

1. Take a large bowl and place the chicken livers in it. Add the lemon juice, vinegar, and 2 tablespoons of olive oil.
2. Season the livers using the cumin, garlic, coriander, salt, bay leaves, pepper, and chilies. Stir the mix and place in the fridge for 1 to 2 hours.
3. Take the livers and place them in a bowl. Reserve the marinade for later.
4. Pour one tablespoon of olive oil and butter in a large skillet and heat over medium heat. Throw in the chopped onion and cook for around 5 minutes. Add the mushrooms and ginger and cook until the mushrooms become tender. Add the chicken livers and raise the heat to medium high. Cook for about 5 minutes, but don't overdo the livers.
5. Add in the marinade and Worcestershire sauce, and simmer for 5 minutes. Finally, pour in the sherry and continue heating.

6. You can serve this dish with your preferred grains or even steamed broccoli.

Serves: 4

Dinner Recipes

Wild Rice Pilaf

This dish contains adequate zinc to boost your vital thyroid functions. Most vegetarians tend to be deficient in this critical mineral, but wild rice is known to contain as much as three times the zinc content of brown rice.

Ingredients:

½ cup wild rice
½ cup brown rice
2 ¼ cups purified water
1/8 tsp powdered cayenne pepper
¾ tsp iodized salt

½ tsp cinnamon
1 ½ tbsp olive oil
2 tbsp gingerroot, peeled and minced
¼ cup raw sunflower seeds
½ cup slivered dry apricots

Instructions:

1. Boil the water in a 2-quart pot, and add salt. Wash the wild rice properly before pouring the wet rice into the boiling water. Minimize the heat level to medium, cover the pot, and then cook for ten minutes.
2. After a 10 minute period, rinse the brown rice and pour it into the same pot. Reduce the heat to medium low. Cover the pot and cook for another 40 minutes.
3. As the rice cooks, sauté the cayenne and cinnamon gently in the vegetable oil using a small pan over low heat. Once the rice is cooked, stir in the spices and apricots.
4. Allow the rice to sit for 1 minute, and then stir in the ginger and sunflower seeds. You can serve the dish warm, at room temperature, or cold.

Serves: 6

Brown Rice with Tomato and Avocado

This is a delicious meal that is not only nutritious but provides you with minerals essential for an underactive thyroid.

Ingredients:

1 cup brown rice

15 cherry tomatoes

1 avocado

2 minced garlic cloves

A few cilantro sprigs

1 squeezed lemon

1 tbsp olive oil

Instructions:

1. Wash the brown rice and pour into a pot of boiling water. Cook for about 30 minutes.
2. Slice the avocado into small pieces. Cut the cherry tomatoes into halves.
3. Combine all the ingredients together in a bowl, then use the mixture to season the rice.
4. Serve on a flat plate.

Serves: 2

Lamb Burger with Kalamata Olives and Mint Gremolata

Lamb meat is a great source of key nutrients, including zinc and vitamin B12.

Ingredients:

1 ½ pounds ground lamb

1/3 cup Kalamata olives, chopped

8 tbsp mint, freshly chopped

1 tbsp organic extra virgin olive oil

½ tsp Celtic sea salt

½ tsp organic dried oregano

¼ cup parsley, freshly chopped

½ tsp freshly ground black pepper

1 organic lemon zest

Instructions:

1. Prepare the gremolata first. Mix the garlic, mint, lemon juice, lemon zest, and parsley together and set it aside.
2. Set the grill or grill-pan on a medium-high heat.
3. Take a large bowl and mix the lamb, oregano, pepper, salt, and olives together. Form ½ inch thick patties. If you are using a grill/ grill pan, heat the burgers for about 4 minutes on each side.
4. When the burgers are done, serve with the gremolata.

Serves: 6

German Rouladen

Ingredients:

24 oz flank steak

2 tbsp butter

2 ½ cups beef stock

2 organic onions

8 tsp mustard

6 slices uncured smoked bacon

4 kosher pickles

Instructions:

1. Take a sharp knife and slice the flank steak into thin filets – about three inches wide and a quarter inch thick.
2. Cut the pickles lengthwise into thin slices.
3. Place the filets of steak on a working surface and apply mustard on them. Top each filet with slices of bacon, pickles and onion. Then roll the steak strip tightly from one end to the other and hold in place with a toothpick.
4. Place a skillet over medium heat and add the butter.
5. Place the steak rolls in the skillet, and cook each side for about two minutes, until they brown.
6. Pour the beef stock into the skillet, cover it, and allow to simmer for about an hour.
7. Serve.

Serves: 6

Lima Bean Hummus

This hummus snack is a simple dish that low in fat and high in tyrosine, which is good for the thyroid. You can have this for dinner if you are alone and don't want to spend too much time preparing something elaborate.

Ingredients:

1 can lima beans

1/3 cup lemon juice

2 cloves garlic, minced

½ tsp ground cumin

Salt to taste

1 tbsp paprika

¼ cup parsley leaves, minced

Instructions:

1. Place all the above ingredients (except the parsley and paprika) in a blender and blend into a puree.
2. Remove the mixture from the blender, place in a bowl and mix in the parsley leaves. Put it in the refrigerator for a couple of hours.
3. Garnish with the paprika. You can serve it with chopped veggies like celery or carrots.

Serves: 2

Vegetable Soup

Ingredients:

1 onion, finely chopped
2 carrots, grated
2 tbsp extra virgin olive oil
1 leek, finely chopped

1 organic vegetable stock cube
4 new potatoes, grated
1 can flageolet beans, drained
Salt and pepper to taste

Instructions:

1. Pour one tablespoon of olive oil into a pot and sauté the onions. Cook on medium heat for about 4 minutes.
2. Toss in the grated carrots and potatoes and cook for another 5 minutes. Then add in the chopped leek and heat for about 3 minutes, until the veggies are *al dente*.
3. Mix the vegetable stock with one liter of boiled water, and then pour it into the pot. Once the mixture has boiled, remove the pot from the heat and puree the mix slowly in a blender.
4. After blending it to your preference, pour the puree back into the pot and place over low heat. You can season with some salt and pepper to taste.
5. Once the puree starts boiling, pour in the Flageolet beans and cook for 2 more minutes. Turn off the heat and allow the food to sit for a couple of minutes.
6. Serve.

Serves: 2

Slow Cooker Black Bean Soup

Here's another great recipe for a healthy thyroid. Since we're dealing with beans, you know you're going to have to soak them overnight, so preparation must start early. Other than that, it's a sumptuous dish.

Ingredients:

8 oz dried organic black beans

2 cups organic chicken broth

½ tsp organic ground cumin

½ tbsp organic chili powder

½ tsp organic garlic powder

½ tsp organic hot sauce

½ tsp organic cayenne pepper

½ tsp ground black pepper

Instructions:

1. Drain the water from the soaked beans, then rinse them out.
2. Place the beans and chicken broth in a slow cooker. Add the cumin, hot sauce, chili powder, cayenne pepper and garlic powder to season the food as it cooks.
3. Raise the heat to high for about 2 ½ hours. Lower the heat to low and cook for two more hours.

Serves: 4

Thai Beef Salad

This is a simple Thai meal with a great combination of ingredients.

Ingredients:

24 oz. grass-fed flank steak

3 organic radishes

1 clove organic garlic

1 cup organic cabbage, shredded

1 tbsp organic palm sugar

½ piece organic carrot

1 tbsp fish sauce

4 tbsp chopped organic cilantro

½ oz. toasted and chopped organic peanuts

½ organic cucumber

1 ½ tsp sriracha chili paste

2 organic scallions, medium sized

1 oz. rice noodles

3 tbsp fresh lime juice

1/3 cup chopped organic tomato

2 tbsp organic almond oil

1/3 cup diced mangoes

½ sesame oil

4 cups mixed baby greens

Salt and pepper to taste

Instructions:

1. Prepare the dressing first. Put the lime juice, minced garlic, palm sugar, fish sauce, almond oil, sriracha, sesame oil, and 1 tablespoon of filtered water in a bowl and whisk together. Set aside as you work with the rest of the ingredients.
2. Use the salt and pepper to season the beef. Then sear the beef on a large skillet, preferably 2 to 3 minutes for each side or until medium rare.
3. Put the meat aside for a couple of minutes and then slice it into thin strips. Toss the meat with the dressing (2 to 3 tablespoons).
4. Take a large bowl and combine the left over salad ingredients (minus the peanuts) with the dressing. Make sure everything is coated well.
5. Put the salad on plates, top off with the beef strips, and then sprinkle the chopped peanuts over it.
6. Serve.

Serves: 4

Herb Roasted Turkey Tenderloin

Ingredients:

32 oz. pasture-raised turkey tenderloin	2 tbsp apple cider vinegar
2 organic shallots	¼ tsp freshly ground black pepper
1 cup organic free range chicken broth	½ tsp Celtic sea salt
½ cup dry white wine	1 tbsp extra virgin olive oil
2 tbsp fresh tarragon	

Instructions:

1. Preheat the oven to 400° F.
2. Coat the inner surface of a large baking dish with oil.
3. Use black pepper and salt to season the turkey, and then place it into the baking dish.
4. Chop the shallots and arrange them on the turkey.
5. Mix the wine, vinegar, broth and chopped tarragon in a small bowl. Pour the mixture all over the turkey.
6. Roast the turkey in an oven for 40 minutes or until it reads 160° F on a meat thermometer.
7. Set the turkey aside for 10 minutes then cut it into ½" thick slices.
8. Serve.

Serves: 4

Lentil Stew

This is a great meal packed with protein and healthy spices. It is also filling and quite inexpensive.

Ingredients:

1 cup lentils

1 tbsp coconut oil

2 tomatoes

½ tsp ground turmeric

1 onion

2 cups filtered water

2 cloves crushed garlic

1 tsp garam masala

1 tsp chopped ginger

Salt and pepper

1 chopped red chili

Instructions:

1. In a pan, heat the coconut oil and sauté the chopped onion, chili, garlic and ginger.
2. Rinse and drain the lentils. Once the onion turns golden brown, add the lentils and garam masala, and sauté for 1 more minute.
3. Add water and chopped tomatoes, bring to a boil, and then reduce the heat.
4. Place the lid over the pan and let it simmer for 40 minutes.
5. Remove the pan from the heat and add the turmeric.
6. This lentil stew can be eaten with brown rice.

Serves: 4

Conclusion

I am reminded of a quote by the legendary Mark Twain, who once said, "The only way to keep your health is to eat what you don't want, drink what you don't like, and do what you'd rather not." In today's world, it is now easier and much more fun to stay healthy, what with all the healthy and delicious meals available. It is the doing part that you have to set your mind to, because without the will to change your lifestyle for the better, even the healthiest meals will not help you.

Now that you have read through this book, you have the information that you need to tackle hypothyroidism as effectively as possible. You now understand more about its causes and symptoms, and the factors that put you at risk.

We have seen just how a good exercise regimen can make a difference in controlling your weight gain and improving your energy levels. Even more importantly, your mental state is also given a boost, considering how depression can easily set in when dealing with this disease.

I'm sure you will enjoy trying out all the recipes provided in this book. Each breakfast, lunch and dinner can now be a fun adventure to be savored — and most of these recipes are pretty easy and don't eat up too much of your time. So just give these natural remedies a chance and you will be amazed at how your health will improve. The progress may take time for some people, but rest assured that the benefits will come.

Finally, if you enjoyed this book, then I'd like to ask you for a favor, would you be kind enough to leave a review for this book on Amazon? It'd be greatly appreciated!

Thank you and good luck!